Tight, Tone, and Trim:

How to get rid of Cankles, Bat Wings, Thunder Thighs, and Muffin Tops. And much, much more!

By

Jack Witt

With illustrations by

Kaitlin Howell

Table of Contents

Part I

Part II

Part III

Introduction

Today we live in a very fast-paced, technologically advanced, rapid-fire Information Age. It's hard to find time for oneself and close friends and family, let alone get to the gym for a workout and cook a healthy meal afterwards. The workweek and commute times are getting longer, and it seems like social networking is eating up a lot of our time, creating empty connections and unnecessary distractions. Add this all together, and you get lots of barriers to health and wellness that we must acknowledge and overcome.

In this book I try to turn back the clock to a simpler, more innocent time with retro- looking, 1950's/1960's illustrations, humorous anecdotes, and a light-hearted atmosphere regarding exercise, nutrition and motivation. It's my aim to harness everything I've learned in my ten years as a health and fitness coach to people of all ages, sizes, and personalities, and to create some simple steps and techniques to help you understand and take charge of your health and well being, while having fun doing it!

I've always felt that fitness and health doesn't have to be overly serious, it doesn't have to be complicated and tedious; it can be a part of your life, not consuming your life. I'm not a super athletic person naturally (I've had to develop that), and when I was growing up in school I was a bit of a class clown, more into music and being in a rock band than playing sports and being a popular jock.

That said, o-happy days are here again, folks, and I'm gonna "sock it to you" with unique and uncomplicated methods for keeping yourself motivated and "bird is the word" on how your food management doesn't have to be rocket science. You'll get some very specific exercise instructions on how to get rid of those "radioactive" common problem areas on the human body, and you'll look and feel terrific as a result!

So enjoy my companion books; *"Cut, Cool & Confident: How to get rid of Beer Belly, Chicken Legs, Wimp Arms, & Man Boobs"* and *"Tight, Tone & Trim: How to get rid of Cankles, Bat Wings, Thunder Thighs, & Muffin Tops"*. E-book versions featuring full color illustrations are available at https://www.amazon.com/author/jackwitt at a discounted price.

Cheers,

Jack Witt
Health and Fitness Coach

SMEFADSAI

I proclaim today as the first day of the rest of your life! Roll out the banners, ticker tape, and marching bands because you are on your way to a brighter tomorrow. You know life is short and it goes by quickly. You know it's never too late to change. You know you have so much untapped potential inside of you.

So today I want you to make a pact with yourself that there's no more looking back, no more being stuck in the present and staring at that face and that body in the mirror, that you simply are not connecting with. I'm yelling at you now, at the top of my lungs, so your inner child baby thing can hear me, "Hey, Real You! Yeah, YOU, way deep down inside, buried and smooshed underneath the façade of this person with Cankles, Bat Wings, Thunder Thighs, and Muffin Tops, it's time to take charge of your fitness, health, and wellness and discover a whole new world of possibilities!"

I truly want you to look your best and be TIGHT, TONE, and TRIM! It's not going to be easy, and there are going to be days where you want to throw in the towel and go back to being the old you that you've grown comfortable with. But I'm sayin' stick with me, folks, 'cause I'm going to show you and I'm going to tell you how to be a fit, happy, and healthy person.

Can you feel it? I call this the process and journey to getting Tight, Tone, and Trim…(sound of a record scratching and/or crickets chirping) "?" Wait a minute; actually, I don't have a special homeopathic, rhyming, or spiritual sounding name for it. So, uh, let's just call it "Stop Making Excuses, Focus, and Do Something About It!" or SMEFADSAI for short.

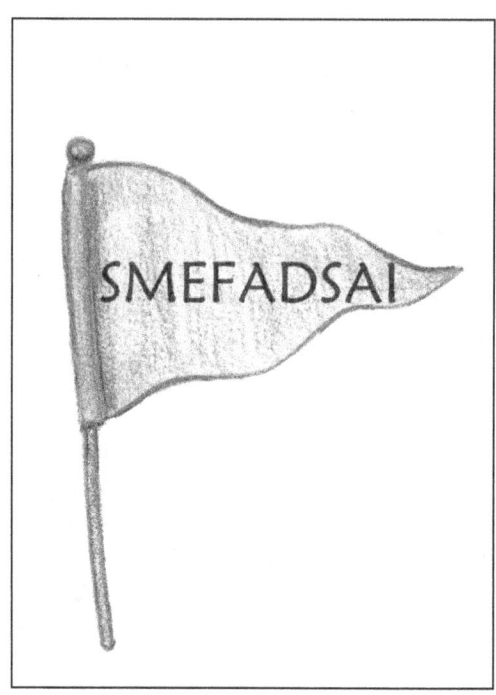

In all my years in the health and fitness industry, helping people of all ages, shapes, and sizes, there are a few common traits or mindsets that I've discovered the most successful clients harness on their journey to a successful SMEFADSAI.

Emotional Intelligence

The first SMEFADSAI is going to be tuning up your emotional intelligence. I live in Hollywood, or, "Hollyweird," as it is sometimes called. Everything here in Tinsel Town revolves around the motion picture industry. It's lights, camera, and action here every day, 24/7. So, I liken emotional intelligence to having the ability to stop the movie that is YOU in your life, step outside of the frame as the actor, YOU, look back at yourself now, as YOU, the director, by slowing the movie frames down and taking notice of how you act and react to certain situations and happenings in your day-to-day life.

In particular, and very importantly, is how you deal with your stressors. Too much stress all at once, or cumulatively over a long period of time, combined with not so good coping habits, can cause chemical, physical, and even hormonal imbalances in your body. These imbalances can lead to all kinds of problems like being overweight, obesity, suppressed immune functions, cancer, high blood pressure, heart attacks, stroke, and death if left unchecked.

Every stressor that we have usually causes a bad habit if not properly dealt with. Some people stress and then eat sweets or salty foods. Some people stress and zone out and watch TV. Whatever it is, take a look at the character of you in your life movie and observe, take notes, and assess how you react and behave in certain situations. Do you like what you are seeing? Or, can you re-write the script to your movie and feature the character of YOU managing stressors better and living a healthier, fit and fulfilled life? This ability is crucial in making the first step towards positive change. Once you make those changes, the Oscar goes to you! (We know; you'd like to thank all the little people!)

It typically takes about 30 to 45 days of consistency to break a bad habit and/or get into a good habit. So I want you to identify a behavior, action, or habit from your life movie that you want to manage first and set up a 30-day action plan to success. Here's how it works: Each day you will do something to counteract that bad habit and/or bring about positive change in your life. For instance, if you come home from work and immediately turn on the TV and zone out with munchies or alcoholic drinks, your 30-day action plan might feature you coming home from work and simply deep breathing for 20 minutes, then stretching for 10 minutes, before you allow yourself to turn on the TV.

Do this for 30 days straight to bring about change. The great thing is, it's like a domino effect - once you break one bad habit there are positive lifestyle changes that will happen in several other areas in your life as a result. How cool is that? You do one positive thing, and a bunch of other little positive things will start happening. You can email me at Jack@GetFitwithWitt.com for a free action plan template. Trust yourself and enjoy your voyage of discovery to a better you.

Faith in Fitness

Another SMEFADSAI is simply having faith in fitness. Can I get a witness?! And it's really more about having faith in the process of fitness and health. You might have faith in God, faith in a person in your life or your family, faith in your community and/or government (well, maybe not government, huh). So you must develop faith in how making positive, healthy changes in your life will help your body, mind, spirit, career, relationships, and circle of family and friends.

I mean, think about it. Have you really ever heard of anybody praising the virtues of being unhealthy and how being unhealthy has helped them with anything in their lives? Well, having faith in fitness and health really isn't taking a big risk. I personally guarantee you that good things will come from it, if you stick to it and make it part of your lifestyle. You've got to have faith! Believe in yourself and who you can become, because if you don't nobody else will.

Get a Little Crazy

Another SMEFADSAI is that you just have to get a little crazy! Yeah, that's right - wacky, insane, and wildly weird about exercise and eating well. As adults we may have a tendency to over think things, dwell on the past, beat ourselves up, or worry about the future. To an extent we must do those things to be realistic about where we're going and what we're doing in our lives

But give yourself permission to just let loose when it comes to your health (in a positive way). Don't expect or demand instant results when starting an exercise program or improving your food intake. Don't dwell on what you are giving up (time and/or money). Don't even worry about what other people think. Just be crazy by trusting and embracing the process, which in turn will stir around those positive brain chemicals called endorphins that will be dancing and prancing around from your healthy and active lifestyle, and in turn will get you "in the zone" of doing the right thing for your body and your mind.

You'll start to hit a stride, and the physically, mentally, and emotionally positive results will start to trickle in and culminate. You'll begin to have extra energy, extra focus and clarity, extra strength, flexibility and range of motion, to get through the normal challenges and obstacles of everyday life. Then the cosmetic changes will start happening and your body will start taking shape, just the way you want it. But notice, I said all this good stuff would start "trickling" in. This isn't a miracle pill or a potion, or a 7-steps-to-change-your-life-in-a-week type of scam. It's a one-day-at-a-time type of "inch-by-inch" approach that is realistic for an everyday, average person like me, and you, and it stays true to your human body, mind, and soul.

Each day will build on the last. Each positive change will snowball into several other positive changes, and a solid foundation will be laid for you to construct yourself into exactly what and who you have always wanted to be. You can't build a house overnight and expect it to be solid, strong, and last a long time. You have to lay the foundation brick by brick. I promise being a little crazy about health and fitness during the process of building YOU day by day does truly work! It might take longer than you want, or it might come sooner than you are ready for. Think about that one...Deep, ay?

Create a Support Network

The last SMEFADSAI is to create a network of support and throw the message out to the Universe every single day that you are adopting a healthier lifestyle and developing into the true you. I'm not talking New Year's Eve, early-January-type resolutions of, "I'm going to get in shape this year," when a few weeks into February all of your health and fitness goals are forgotten. I'm talking true commitment, a whatever-it-takes type of attitude, "This is do or die."

Find family members, and co-workers and friends with whom you can talk to, Facebook, text, tweet, Google Talk, instant message, or Skype (I'm trying to sound tech-savvy here, folks, but half of these will probably be obsolete by the time you read this book) with about what you are doing for your health each day. We all need support and encouragement when getting out of our comfort zone and trying to make positive changes. So use your sphere of influence and your connections to keep you motivated and focused.

You have to throw it out to the Universe each day that you are going to do, or have done, something positive for your body and mind during your transition. No matter how big or small, just keep throwing it out there and throwing it out there. We all know the story of "The Secret" - the Universe will provide back to you; it will supply you with somebody or something that will come into your life to propel and catapult you even further into good fitness, health and wellness. Whatever it turns out to be, embrace it and go with it. You are going to be a different person!

You know, being unhealthy and out of tune with your mind and body is sort of like the flip side of having an addiction problem. People who have addictions will lie, cheat, deceive and steal to keep their habit alive. It's usually not until they have some type of spiritual awakening, or commit to a lifestyle change program, treatment or therapy, that they finally overcome the problem.

Similarly, people who want to take charge of their health and fitness have to treat that process with the same sense of urgency and respect as those trying to shake an addiction. It's a sort of parallel universe; you are actually addicted to non-action, procrastination, fear and neglect of your mind, body, and spirit. I'm coining a new term for this: "Unhealthy-o-holic." So if you can hire a life coach, personal trainer, or professional therapist, do it and do it now!

Time to Get Started

Okay, ladies (and maybe guys if you are reading this), the next section of this book is dedicated to controlling those problem areas of your body: *Cankles*, *Bat Wings*, *Thunder Thighs*, and *Muffin Tops*. Concentrate first on the most severe area of your body, and prioritize the rest from there.

In addition to the directions and exercise plans I'll be laying out for you, you will need to also be doing some type of cardio every other day. This will help with general fat loss throughout your body, including those problem areas. I would recommend at least 30 minutes per day of some type of cardio training. This could be anything from jogging, stationary bike, elliptical, and hiking, to running in place. If you are not sweating and a little out of breath, you are probably performing below the optimal level to create a fitness change. So, make sure your intensity is sufficient, and when 30 minutes starts to feel too easy, increase your time/duration and/or your intensity (i.e. incline on the treadmill, level of difficulty of your hike).

One important rule to remember is how to calculate your maximum heart rate for safety purposes. That formula is 220-your age. For instance, if you are 40 years old, 220-40 = 180, so 180 heartbeats per minute is the upper level of where you should be. If it's anything over this number, you may be doing too much and need to slow down and lessen your time or intensity. Ideally, you should be at about 80% of this number (180 x 80% = 144 beats per minute) to be in the cardio "zone" for an optimal workout. Many cardio machines have sensors that will measure your heart rate, or you can have a fitness trainer or qualified professional calculate your heart rate by taking your pulse from the carotid artery of your neck.

Nutrition Tips and Food Management

Now, one more thing, before we get into the exercises for those problem areas, it's important to talk about your food intake. I always say that about 70% of getting into good shape and being healthy is food management. You can exercise until "the cows come home," but your efforts could be completely erased and nullified by the choices you make on meals and snacks.

What I've learned throughout many years as a health and fitness coach is that if you think you are doing a good job on your food management, you are not. If you think you are doing a great job on your food management, you are only doing a decent job. And, if you think you are doing perfect, you are probably only doing a fairly good job. That's how tough it is to eat properly. Over the past 25-or-so years, portion sizes have gone up something like 600%. Americans eat about 100 pounds more food a year than we did back then. There are more fast food chains and convenience stores all around us, filled with unhealthy and processed foods. We now consume roughly 20% of our daily calories through sugary and fatty beverages (think sodas and Starbucks' white chocolate, mocha-type lattes with whipped cream). All the extra energy from these calories just gets stored as fat in our bodies, because we are also more sedentary.

Creating a perfect storm for overweight and obesity, we work longer hours these days, and commute times are longer than they were 20 years ago. The average American watches around five hours of TV per day. That's not including time on the Internet, surfing the web or watching on-line TV shows or movies, or playing on your smart phone and/or tablet. So, unless you have mastered the art of food management, you risk not burning off enough extra calories to make a substantial impact in your fitness goals. You must become the master of your food and beverage intake.

It's funny, but when you do an on-line search for "diets," you get about 40 million results. I wonder why with that much information right at our fingertips, our fingertips still choose to reach for cookies or pizza?! Over the years I've had clients ask me about crazy diets that involve no carbs, no white foods, higher protein, no fruits or veggies (c'mon does that really sound humanly healthy?), liquids only, raw food only, no eating after 6pm, eating according to your blood type, drinking some type of mother's milk (whose mother I have no idea), eating meat only when the moon is full (okay, not true, but you get the idea). I usually say to them it doesn't have to be rocket science, just stick to the basics and don't over-think it.

Have you ever travelled to another country and wondered why all the people look so thin and still eat normal food, and have dessert? When I went to Paris and observed all the locals still eating their desserts and bread while remaining overall pretty thin-bodied, I observed it's because they eat normal portions and they don't eat very many processed foods. Most things are fresh baked and prepared daily. They probably walk around a lot more than we do here in the States, burning more calories, but I bet they don't have as many gyms as we do. So in regards to dieting, here's one basic down-to-earth strategy: Just focus on what I call your PP (gotcha! No, not that one!): PORTIONS & PROCESSED.

Portions

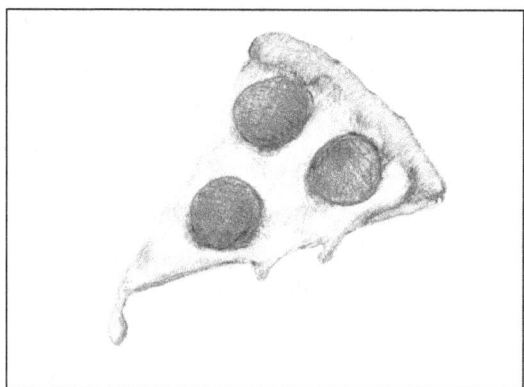

As I mentioned, food portion sizes have gone up drastically in the past few decades. Our bodies just don't require that amount of extra stored energy per meal or snack (which ultimately gets turned into fat on your body). Even if you're eating an organic grilled range free humane certified piece of chicken breast, if it's too large a portion it's just going to get stored as fat.

C'mon, we're not running from Saber Toothed tigers anymore or walking a hundred miles every day, searching for food sources. We're usually stuck in traffic, or lying on the couch, flipping through our 500 cable or satellite channels on our TV's, and/or sitting in front of a computer screen with internet paralysis. Folks, we act like we're pigs at a trough when food is around; we have to remember that food is simply fuel for our bodies and minds.

When you are getting ready to eat, you gotta ask yourself, "Why am I eating this meal?" Is it to provide energy for your work day ahead? Is it to recover after a tough workout? Is it so you have antioxidants to fight off free radicals? Is it for the fiber to help clear out the cholesterol in your body? Whatever the case, each meal and snack you eat should have meaning attached to it.

If you're constantly over-eating and over-indulging, try these tips:

> When you are hungry, wait 10 minutes before eating and then chew your food slowly. It takes 20 minutes for your mind to tell your stomach you are full.

> Drink a glass of water before eating to make you feel fuller.

> Eat foods that are less calorie-dense (i.e. fruits, vegetables).

> Don't eat 1/4 of whatever is on your plate. "Save that for the Devil," as they say.

> Don't keep junk food in the house/apartment. This is a rule that I live by. Most cravings aren't strong enough to make you get in the car and drive down to the store to pick up some junk food. So, if it's not in the house/apartment, then you won't have it. And, by George, amazingly, you'll be thinner and leaner in no time!

In regards to portions, a very simple and easy way to stay on track with your food portions is by using the "eyeball method" to compare proper portion sizes to something that you are familiar with, like a computer mouse or a set of dice.

Familiarize yourself with these and for the rest of your life you'll never have to guess again:

Meat

> 3 ounces of meat: deck of cards or palm of your hand without your fingers

Breads, cereals, rice and pasta

> An average bagel: a hockey puck

> A medium potato: a computer mouse

> 1 cup of rice or pasta: size of your fist

> 1 cup dried cereal: a large handful

Dairy

> 1-1/2 ounces natural cheese: 4 dice

Fats, Oils and Sweets

> 1/2 cup of ice cream: a tennis ball

> 1 teaspoon butter, salad dressing, peanut butter or mayonnaise: one die (dice)

FYI: one tablespoon = 3 teaspoons

Fruit

> 1 medium fruit: a tennis ball

> 1 cup of fruit: a baseball

> 1/2 cup chopped fruit: 15 marbles

Vegetables

> 1 cup lettuce: 4 leaves

> 1 cup vegetables (chopped): a fist

> 1.2 cup vegetables (chopped): light bulb

Processed Foods

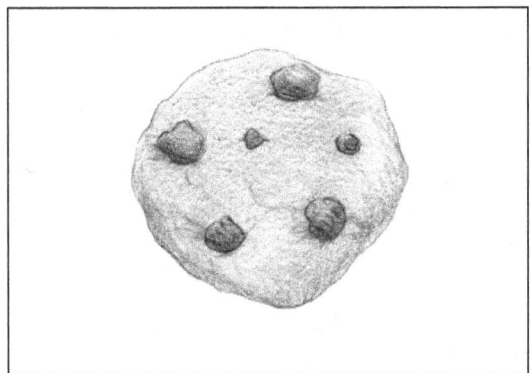

Cheap to manufacture, easy, quick and addictive to eat, but causing disease, depression and obesity like nobody's business. Wean yourself off of eating processed foods and you'll look and feel awesome! Here's how: Start by choosing one day a week where you have absolutely no processed foods. Maybe it would be easier to do it on a weekend if you are less busy and stressed. Remember, only wholesome, natural foods with no extra additives, hormones, or ingredients you can't pronounce. At the end of the day, make it a point to write down how you feel. Do you have more energy? Are you more focused? Do you have less heartburn? Then the next morning, make it a point to document how you feel when you wake up. Are you more alert? Are you more energized? Are you ready to seize the day?

After you have weaned yourself completely off of processed foods, one day a week for 4 weeks in a row, then try to add another day of the week where you are processed-foods free. Yep, that's two complete days per week. You can do it! Keep a journal of how you feel each day. Also, be alert as to how other things in your life might be changing. Are people around you treating you better? Are you more effective and efficient at work? Are you accomplishing more in your personal and professional life? Do you have a more positive attitude in general?

Keep progressing by adding in an additional day of the week that you are processed-foods free. You will be amazed at how your body starts changing for the better. You'll even notice your joints feeling better and having more range of motion! Our body just wasn't meant to have all that crap in it, it doesn't know what to do with it, so it builds up as fat and/or becomes a breeding ground for cancer cells. As they say in Costa Rica, "Pura Vida," which means live the "Pure Life." You'll virtually become a different person without processed foods and experience what the Ticos (local Costa Ricans) mean by that phrase.

Did you know? In the 1960's food manufacturers began using High Fructose Corn Syrup (HFCS) to sweeten foods because it was cheap to use. Since then, as the usage of this sweetener has increased, so has the obesity rate in the USA. HFCS contains elements that inhibit insulin from being released to lower our blood sugar levels. Bottom line, that's real bad.

So remember, if you don't approach your food management with complete urgency, dedication and focus, you absolutely will not succeed in your fitness goals. I came across a poster once that sums it all up, "Anyone can work out for an hour, but to control what goes on your plate the other 23 hours…that's the hard work." Chew on that!

One last thing before we get to the exercises for your *Cankles, Thunder Thighs, Bat Wings, and Muffin Tops*: always check with your doctor before you start any new workout or diet program. It's also a good idea to have a certified and experienced fitness trainer to supervise at least your first few workouts to make sure you are using proper form and not risking injury to yourself. And, always warm up properly before starting your program.

So with all of that said, let's get you TIGHT, TONE, and TRIM! Flap those bat wings, and turn the page now.

Cankles

How to get rid of and prevent CANKLES, also known as Chubby Ankles, Stovepipe Legs, Tree Trunks, Softball Coach Butchy Calves, Sausage Legs, and Capri Pant Killers.

Cankles are basically a lack of a defined indent where your calves meet your ankles, which can also be described as short thick ankles with no shape. I've heard it described, "It's like my calf muscle merged with my foot and cut out the middleman." Sometimes it's hereditary and/or it may be excess body fat that deposits itself in your calf/ankle area instead of your thighs, hips, or belly. Some other causes could be abnormal water retention, tendinitis, pregnancy edema, or an Achilles tendon injury that brings on chronic swelling.

They can also be the result of a low muscular attachment of the gastrocnemius muscle (the convex, bulgy part of the calf) and a shorter soleus muscle (the muscle just above your Achilles tendon) so that the main belly of the calf is not as differentiated. There are doctors who advertise liposuction for this problem area (not recommended for the budget-conscious), and some people have been known to do crazy things like applying Preparation H hemorrhoid cream to the affected area and then wrapping it with an Ace bandage (not recommended for anybody that's sane).

Cankles, like other problem areas that I will be addressing in this book, can't be solely spot trained. Spot training means you pick an area on your body and just do exercises for that part, hoping it will shrink. This is a common mistake when people want to slim down their tummy and get those six pack abs. They'll do sit ups for an hour hoping that somehow the body will only suck the fat from the area being worked out.

It usually doesn't work like this. That's because when you exercise, your fat cells are triggered by adrenaline to release fat, but some cells are more stubborn than others, and that affects the pattern in which weight is lost. Your genes determine this pattern. And that pattern may make you lose the fat in your thunder thighs before your cankles. But eventually, you will lose the fat somewhere, and the more consistent you are with your exercising and your healthy eating, you'll eventually become tight, tone, and trim, everywhere!

Now, you'll need to get going on a cardio routine, as I've already mentioned, for a complete body calorie/fat burn. Simultaneously, we will still have focused resistance/weight-bearing types of exercises to do for each problem area to help chisel away more definition, as the fat from the cardio is melting away.

Here are some great exercises that you can do to ship-shape-up your calf and ankle area, in addition to doing your cardio and eating healthy:

Standing Calf Raise

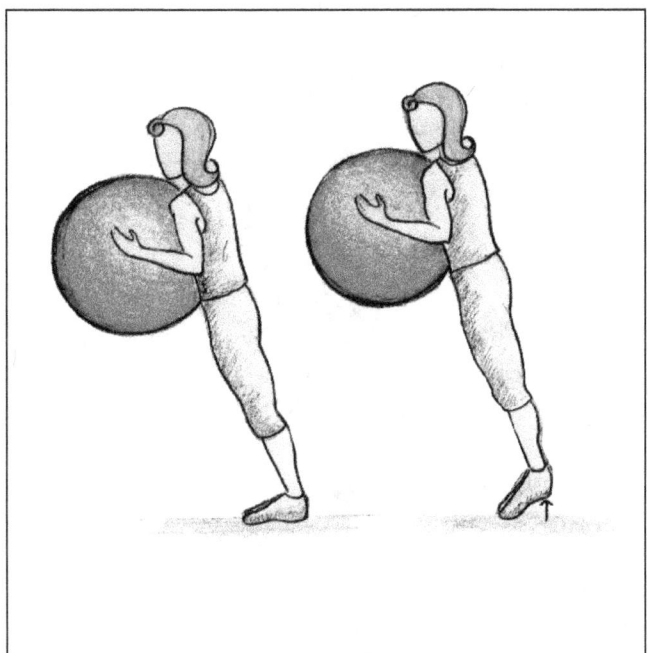

1) Your starting position is going to be to standing with your feet about hip-width apart, leaning against a stability ball on a wall, or standing on the edge of a step with your heels hanging off, while holding onto something secure.

2) Flex your calves by pushing off the balls of your feet and raising your heels up in air (so that you're standing on your toes).

3) Lower your heels back down, feel the stretch in your calves, and repeat. I'd recommend three sets of 20 repetitions.

4) Remember to keep your knees slightly bent throughout this movement to prevent any knee strain. Traditionally this exercise is done with feet pointing straight ahead; however, you can change the emphasis of the workout by pointing your feet out (which works your inner calf more) or in towards each other (works your outer calf).

Seated Calf Raise with Dumbbells

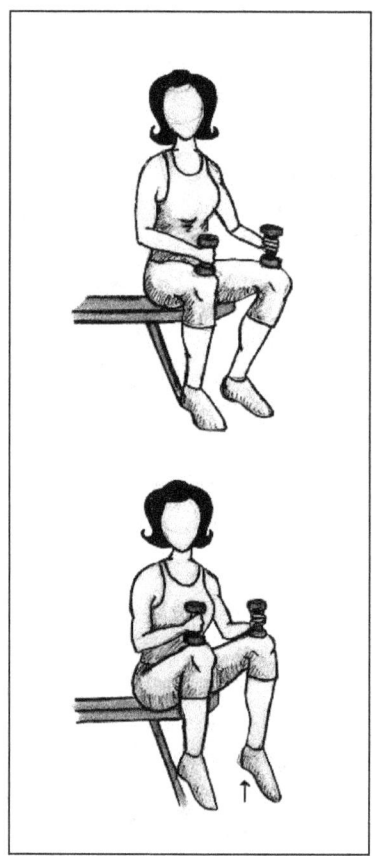

     1) Sit in an upright position on a bench or stability ball with your knees bent at 90 degrees and feet flat on the floor. Place the balls of your feet on a step or any kind of ledge (heels should be off of the step). Then place a dumbbell or some kind of weight on top of each thigh just behind your knees.

     2) Raise your heels up by pushing off the balls of your feet.

     3) Lower your heels to below the level of the step and feel the stretch.

     4) Remember to sit upright with your back and your head straight in a neutral position. I'd recommend three sets of 20 repetitions.

Jump Rope (basic two feet version)

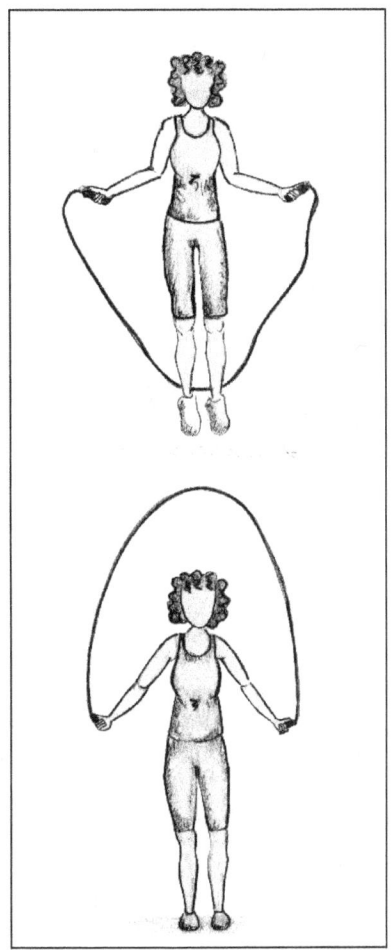

1) Start with the jump rope in each hand.

2) Jump off the ground and start swinging the jump rope around to the front of your body and then under your feet and back around again.

3) Complete three sets of 50 jumps. When you feel comfortable with this exercise, try doing it backwards.

Jumping Jacks

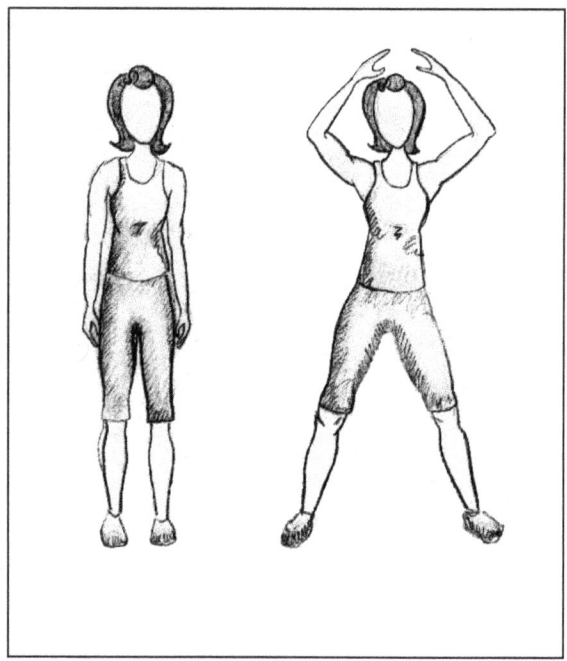

1) Start by standing with your legs side by side and your arms down straight by your sides.

2) In one motion jump and spread your legs out to the side (laterally) while your arms raise out (laterally) and up over your head (abduct).

3) Land back down in this position, and then return to the starting position and repeat for three sets of 50.

Walking Backwards on a Treadmill

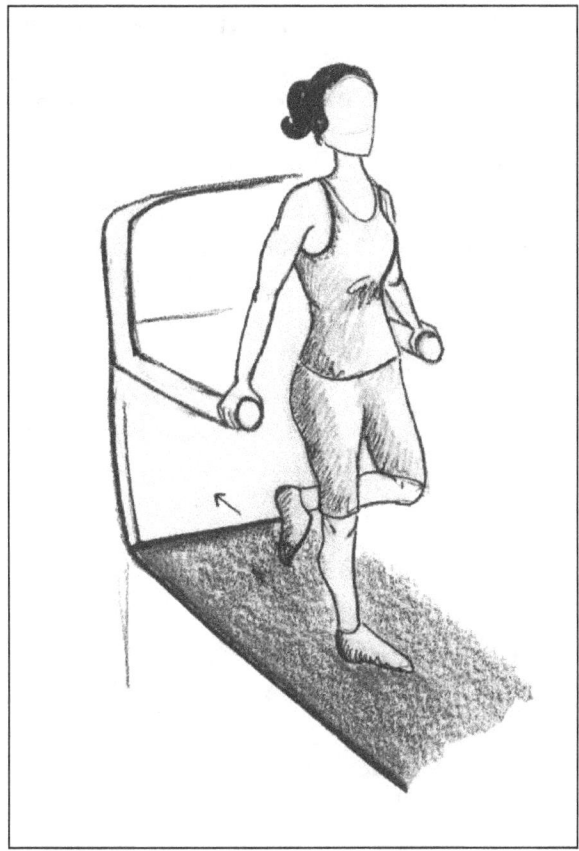

1) Stand on the sides of the treadmill facing forward at first (straddling the belt).

2) Turn the treadmill on and set the speed at a safe number (I'd recommend two to three to start, but every treadmill is calibrated differently, so use extra precaution and start slow).

3) Holding onto the rails, slowly turn around and face away from the console while using a toe-ball-heel stride to walk. Keep holding the rails until you feel comfortable with your balance.

4) Let go of the rails when you are ready, and pump your arms as you walk backwards. Don't lean forward too much, or backward too much. Keep a somewhat erect posture while walking backwards.

5) Do this for 10 minutes to start, and gradually add time (duration) to your workout.

Some additional tips for getting rid of and preventing Cankles:

> Cut down on salt to avoid additional water retention in your ankles.

> Elevate your feet to drain fluid away from your ankles.

> Avoid long periods of inactivity to cut down on water retention.

> Cut down on alcohol consumption to avoid water retention.

Bat Wings

How to get rid of BAT WINGS, also referred to as Ooogies, Lunch Lady Arms, Bingo Wings, Flabby Arms, and Jiggly Arms.

Bat wings - the name used to describe the loose skin that dangles when you extend out your arms. In fact, when you shake your arms, it just might create a wind gust! This happens mostly to women, and many wish they could just snip off some of that arm fat. If this is you, it's time to roll up your sleeves (and your bat wings) and get down to work with exercises for the backs of your arms.

Bat wings can be caused by weight gain, or even weight loss. As we get older, our skin starts losing its ability to snap right back after weight loss. It's just not as elastic. Also, many women, as they age, begin to store a lot of body fat around their triceps, creating that bat wing look.

It's important to note that your triceps muscle (back of your arm) is two-thirds of your arm's muscle, so you've really got to give it proper attention and not just focus on the bicep (front of your arm).

Do this arm routine every other day in addition to your cardio and healthy eating, and say goodbye to the arm flab factor!

Diamond Pushups

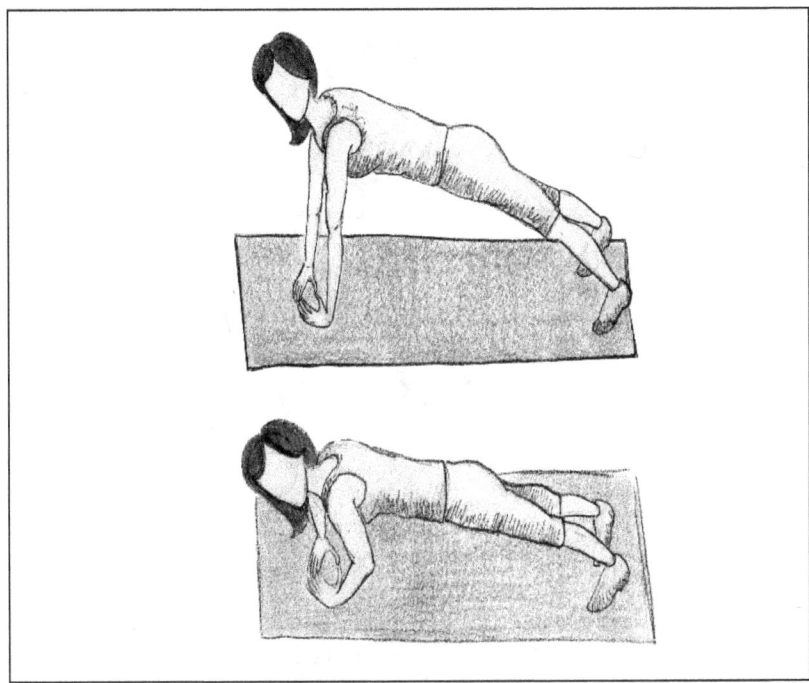

1) Lie face down on the floor and place your hands in the center of your chest to form a diamond shape (kind of a triangle type shape) with your index fingers and thumbs. Your feet should be at hip width with your toes on the floor. (You may do an alternate style instead, which means your knees can be on the floor while your feet/toes are up.)

2) Extend your elbows (straighten your arms) and raise your body off of the floor.

3) Lower your entire body (legs, hips, trunk, and head) three to seven inches from the floor.

4) Return to the starting position by extending at the elbows and pushing your body up.

5) Remember to keep your body straight and avoid sticking your butt up in the air. Draw your naval into your spine. Never fully lock out your elbows and avoid hyperextension of your back, while keeping your head in a neutral position.

6) Do three sets of 15 repetitions

Triceps Bench Dip

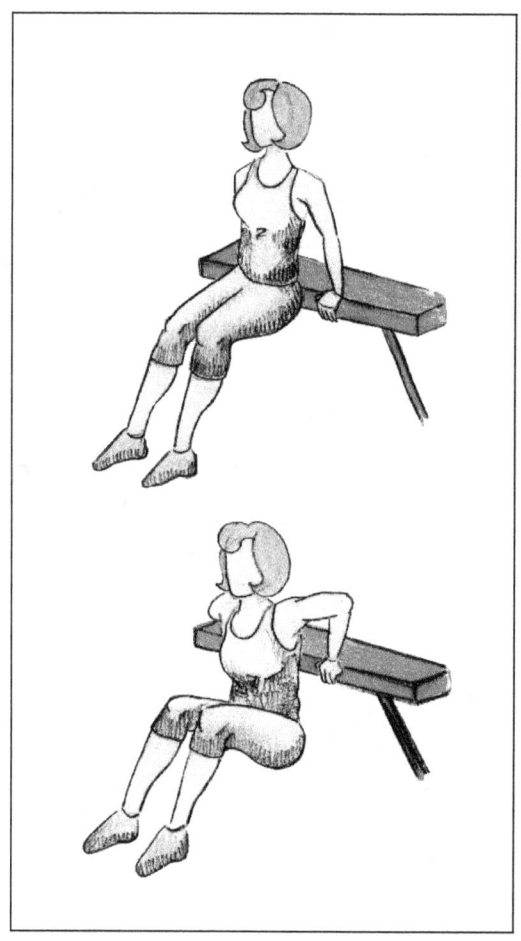

1) Start by placing your hands on a bench or the edge of a secure chair, and your feet on the ground with your legs semi straight. Your butt should not be on the surface.

2) Now flex (bend) your arms and lower yourself down with your butt going towards the floor. Your arms should end up bent at about 90 degrees.

3) Return back to the starting position and extend (straighten) your arms.

4) Do three sets of 15 repetitions if you can. If it feels too difficult, just do a few (safety first) and work your way up. The more straightened your legs are, the greater the level of difficulty.

DB Overhead Triceps Extension

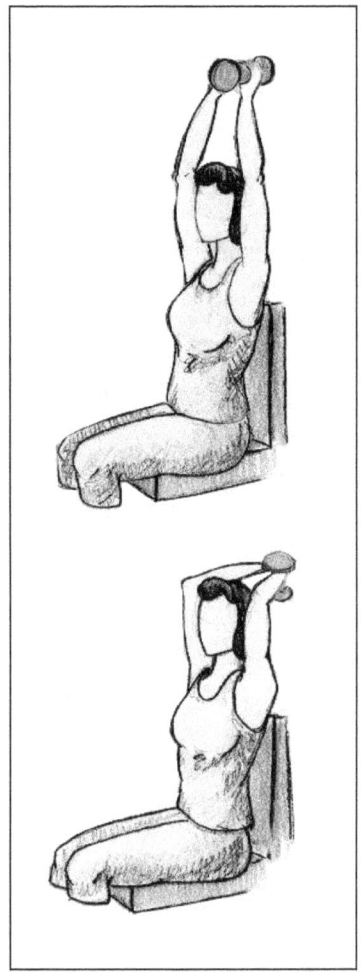

1) Sit with your feet shoulder width apart in an upright position on a bench with back support, or a stability ball.

2) Clasp your hands around a dumbbell and lift it above your head so your palms are up and your arms are extended almost straight.

3) Stabilize your shoulders and lower the weight down in the back of your head, moving only at the elbow joint until your forearm is parallel to the floor. Keep your elbows pointing forward throughout the movement.

4) Extend your arms straight back again, bringing the weight up above your head. Remember to keep your back straight and your head in a neutral position. Don't flare your elbows out during the movement.

5) Do three sets of 15 repetitions with a weight that is challenging, but not too heavy that it would cause you to break form.

Bicep Curl with a Fit Band

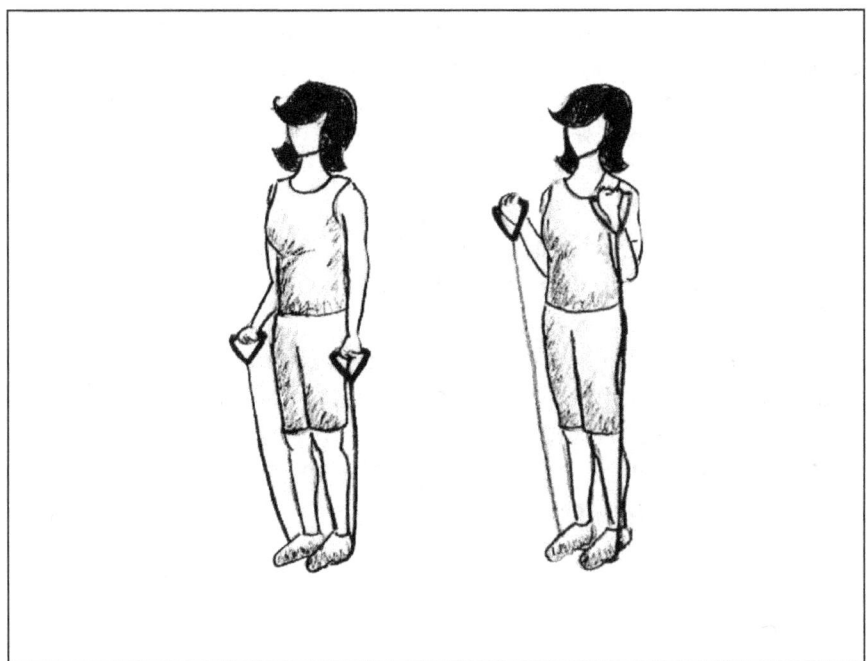

1) With your fit band laid out on the floor, stand with your feet shoulder width apart on the band.

2) Grasp the handles with an underhand grip (palms facing forward) and hang your arms down at your side. Elbows should be close to your body.

3) Curl up with the handles to right around shoulder level. Keep your elbows close to your sides throughout the entire range of motion.

4) Return back down by extending and straightening your arms at the elbow joint.

5) Remember to keep your back and head straight in a neutral position throughout the curl. Your shoulders should be stabilized by squeezing your shoulder blades together just slightly. Only the elbow joint should be moving.

6) Do three sets of 15 repetitions. If the resistance is too much, just step on the band with one foot while your other foot/leg is behind it firmly on the floor.

Some additional tips on preventing and curing "Bat Wings":

>   When getting up from a chair or seat that has arm rests, use a little bit more of your arm and shoulder muscles instead of your legs by pushing off the arm rests slowly while rising. This will engage your triceps primarily and over time will help to keep the back of your arms in shape.

>   When you are washing your hair, spend a little extra time with that up and down movement of your arm at the elbow joint while you are shampooing to engage the triceps muscles.

>   Pinch the back of your arm periodically each week to get a feel and measure of how much fat is in your bat wing. Visualize it becoming less and less, and monitor how much you have improved each week by measuring the distance with your middle finger from the end of your index finger to where the pinched fat ends.

Thunder Thighs

How to get rid of THUNDER THIGHS, also known as Saddlebags and Wobbly Thighs.

Okay, gals, I know it's unfair that women tend to deposit much of their fat on the thighs, hips, and butt. Of course, this used to be an advantage thousands of years ago for pre- and post-natal women during times of famine and drought. But our cave dwelling days are over, and that extra fat padding is unwanted and just causes frustration. (And, if your legs rub together when you walk and make a sound, it's enough to make you want to hide in a cave.)

Let's take action right now and get those Thunder Thighs under control. It's all about slimming down your inner, (adductor muscles) and outer (abductor muscles), thighs. You'll also want to incorporate some front thigh (quadriceps) muscles and back of the leg (hamstring) muscles, too, for a completely toned-up look. And let's not forget the bootie (glutes), which works together with all your thigh and leg muscles for movement.

I want you to do these exercises at least three times per week for your thighs/legs/butt/hips, along with a daily cardio (at least 30-minute) routine for all around fat loss (jogging, stationary bike, elliptical etc.) along with healthy eating.

Hip Adductor Raise (inner thighs)

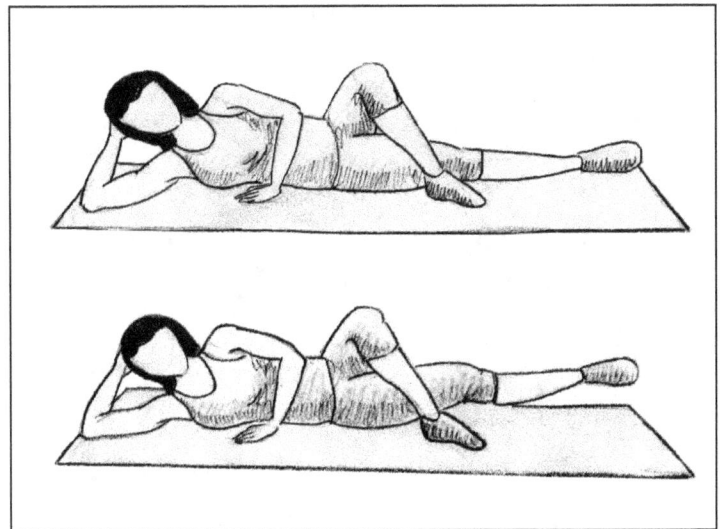

1) Lie on your side and lean up on your elbow. Keeping your bottom leg straight and resting on the floor, wrap your top leg around the bottom leg and place the foot of your top leg on the floor just above the knee of your bottom leg.

2) Pump your bottom leg up and down, still keeping it straight.

3) Repeat for 25 repetitions and then repeat with the other leg, three sets each leg.

Standing Hip Abduction (outer thighs) with a Fit Band

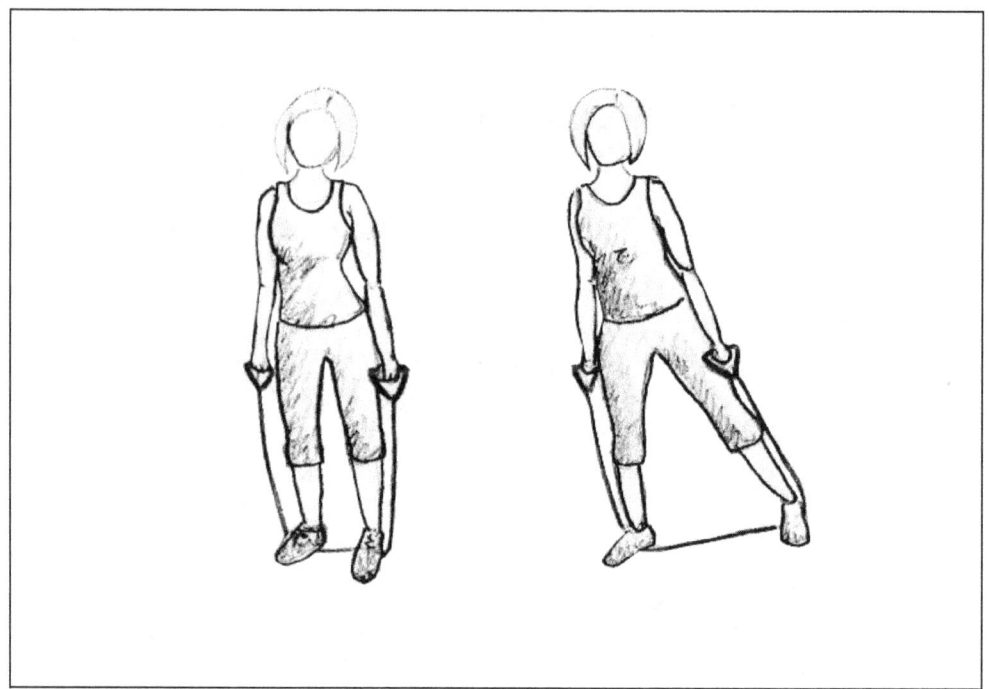

1) Place a fit band (tubing) on the floor and step on it with feet about shoulder width apart.

2) Grab the handles and stand up straight with your arms at your sides.

3) Raise one leg up and out to the side laterally against the fit band to about 45 degrees and then bring it back slowly towards the midline of your body and the starting position.

4) Keep your knee soft on the non moving leg that is doing the standing and balancing.

5) Complete 3 sets of 20 repetitions for each leg.

Stationary Bodyweight Lateral Lunge/Squat

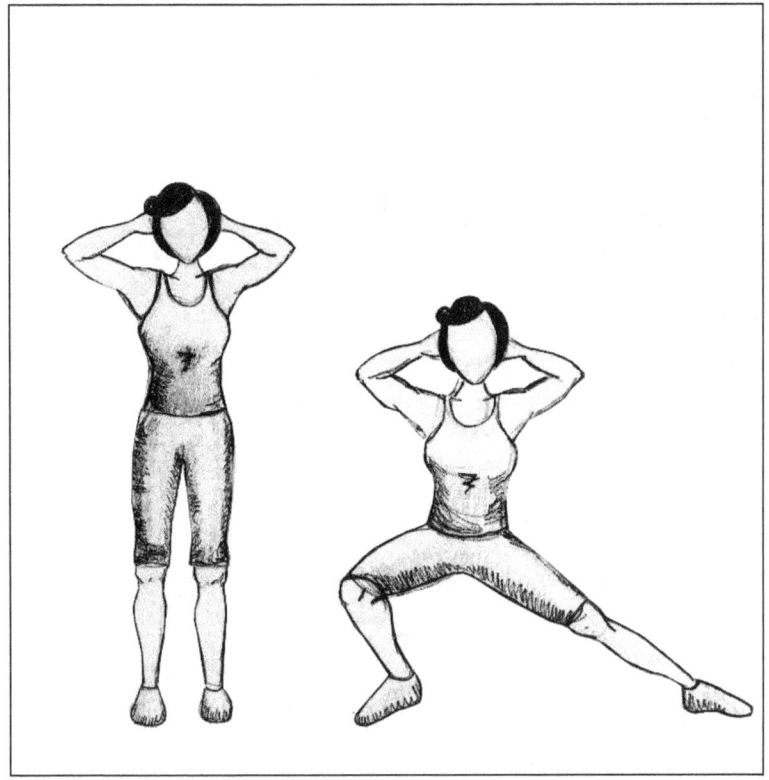

1) Standing upright, place your hands behind your head and position your feet with a moderately wide stance, toes pointing slightly out.

2) Shift your weight and your hip to one side and squat down so that your hip drops down behind that foot and your knee bends.

3) Return to the starting position and repeat the same movement on the other side.

4) Alternate this movement back and forth, completing 50 total repetitions (25 each side) for three complete sets.

5) Remember not to bend over frontward too far; placing unwanted extra pressure on your lumbar.

Lying Hamstring Curl with Stability Ball

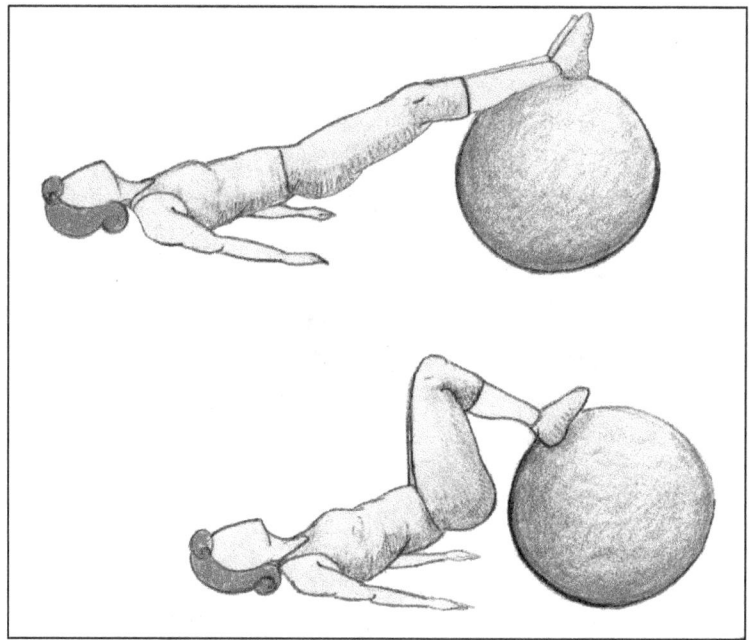

1) Lie on your back, palms down, with your legs straight, resting your heels on top of the stability ball.

2) Raise your butt off the ground and curl your legs by bringing your heels in towards your butt.

3) Return to the starting position, keeping your butt off the ground, and repeat for 25 repetitions. Do three sets.

Fire Hydrants

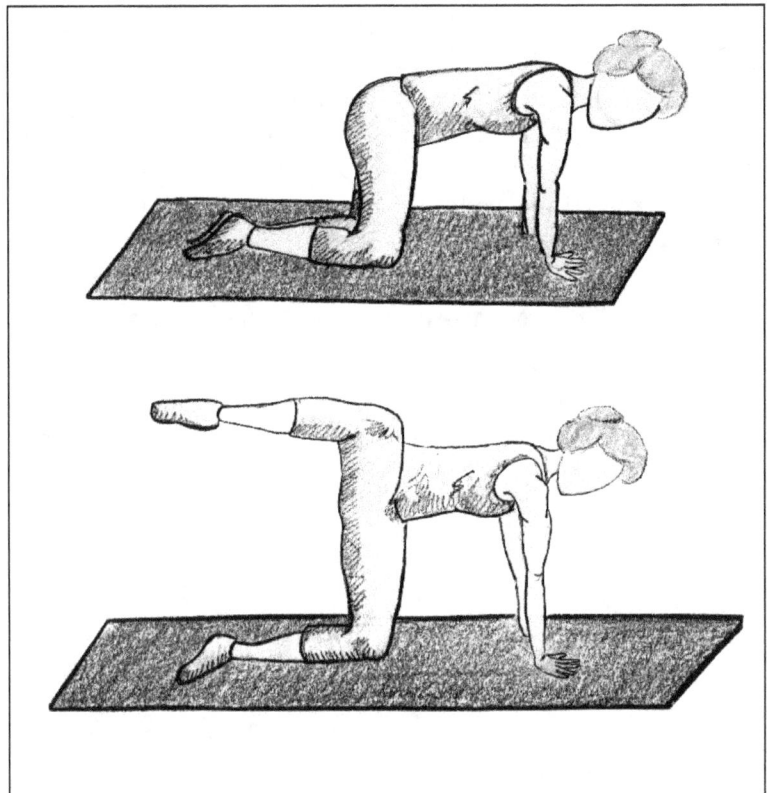

1) Start by kneeling on all fours with your head in a neutral position.

2) Keeping your knee bent, raise one leg up and out to the side. (Think of the movement a dog does with a fire hydrant.)

3) Maintain your posture and balance, and do not lean to the side while doing this exercise. Your back should stay nice and flat.

4) Return back down to the starting position.

5) Do three sets of 20 repetitions each side.

Some additional tips on reducing and getting rid of Thunder Thighs:

> When you're sitting in a chair, squeeze your butt cheeks periodically, and also activate your outer things by moving your legs in and out while your feet stay flat on the floor. For your inner thighs you can squeeze a pillow or a small medicine ball between your legs while sitting.

> Walk more and move more. Get a pedometer and count your steps daily to make sure you are doing enough. The standard minimum is 10,000 steps. Some of my clients use the Fit Bit and the Polar Loop to track all of their daily movements and active choices.

Muffin Top

How to get rid of MUFFIN TOP, also known as Belly Pooch and Fat Tire.

Does your flab spill over the waistband of your pants? That unwanted overhanging fat can occur with low rise pants and midriff tops, and can happen any time you wear a pair of tight pants. It ends up resembling a muffin rising from its paper wrapping. It can be your back fat, stomach fat, love handles, or all of them!

Anytime you have fat in the stomach area, you are at risk for health complications due to its proximity to other organs. A high waist circumference and too much abdominal fat puts you at high risk for Type-2 diabetes, high blood pressure, high cholesterol and heart disease. Women with waist measurements of over 35 inches (88 cm), and men 40 inches (102 cm) are at risk.

To measure your waist circumference, use a tape measure. Start at the top of your hip bone, then bring it all the way around so it's level with your navel. Make sure it's not too tight and that it is parallel with the floor. Don't suck your stomach in too much or hold your breath while measuring it!

Here's some great exercises you can do to "whittle the middle" and get rid of those Muffin Tops!

Ankle Wiggles

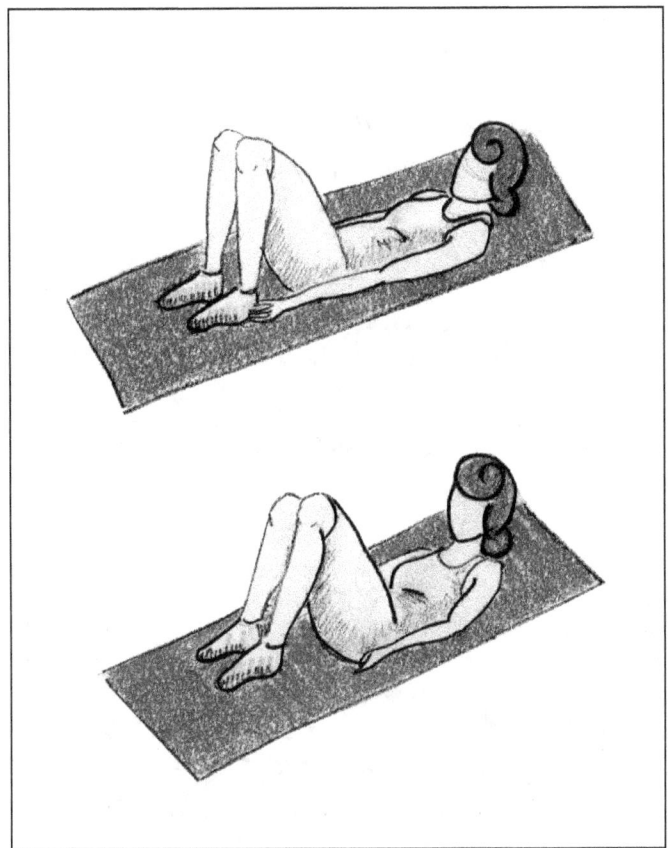

1) Lie on your back, on the floor or a bench, with your knees bent, feet flat on the floor, and your hands at your side. Your head should be in a neutral position with a space between your chin and chest.

2) Raise your head off the floor a few inches while your chin and chest are pointing up towards the ceiling. Contract the abs and raise your rear shoulders off the floor.

3) Reach for your ankle with the hand on the same side and repeat on the other side.

4) Go back and forth for a set of 50 (25 each side) for three sets.

5) Remember to keep your head and shoulder blades up off the floor, enough so that it doesn't place a strain on your neck.

Reverse Crunch Scissor Kicks

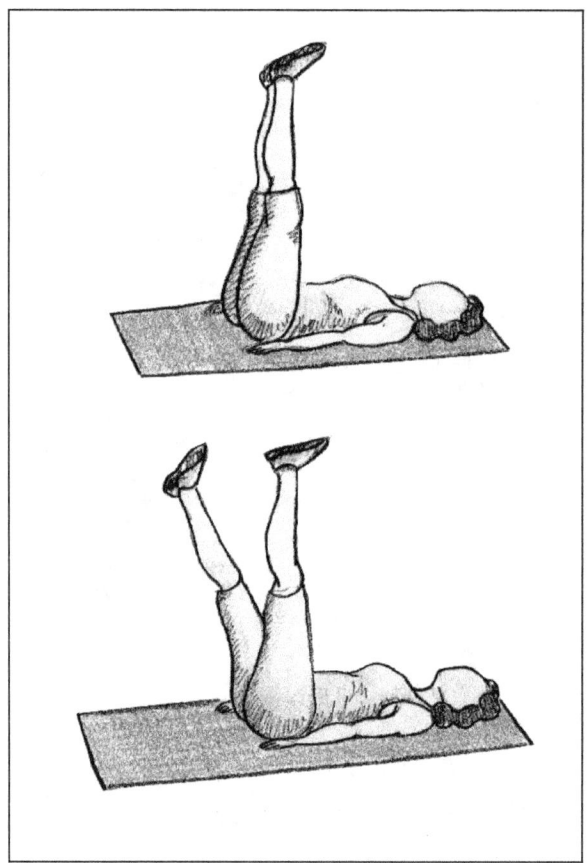

1) Start by lying on your back with arms to your side, palms down, or hands placed under the small of your back for lumbar support. Raise your legs so they are perpendicular to the floor.

2) Lower one leg down almost all the way to the floor or until you are no longer able to keep your lower back neutral to the floor.

3) Lift your leg back up and then repeat with the other leg in a scissor type motion for three sets of 50 repetitions (25 each side).

Lying Side Crunch

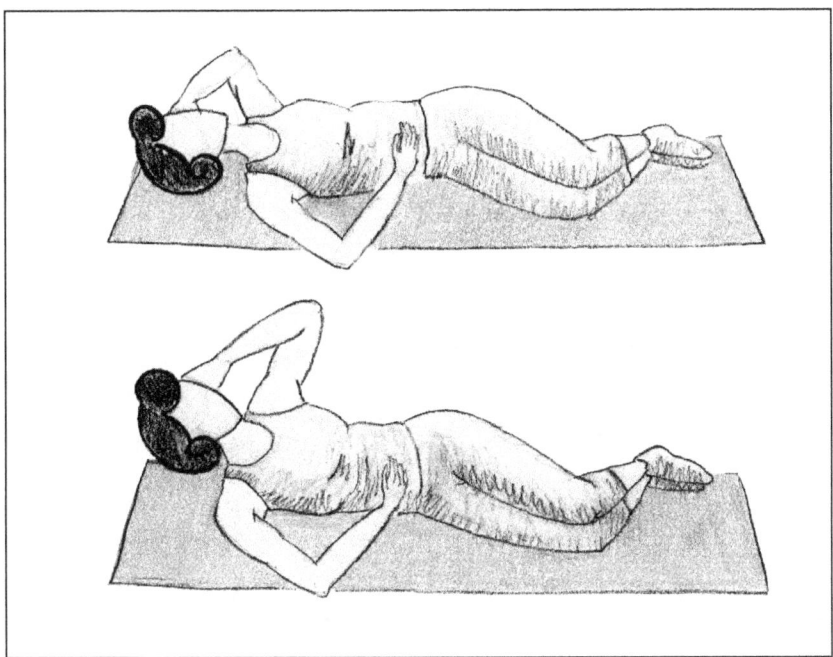

1) Lie with your back on the floor or a bench, with knees bent.

2) Let your knees fall to the right so that your hips are somewhat rotated.

3) Extend your right arm out to the side, straight with palm down, and place your left hand behind your head.

4) Crunch your left side by swinging your left elbow towards your left knee.

5) Do three sets of 20 repetitions. Repeat with the other side.

6) Don't twist excessively; your elbow doesn't need to touch your knee. Simply focus on getting a contraction of your side ab muscles above your hip and below your rib cage.

Cobra on Floor

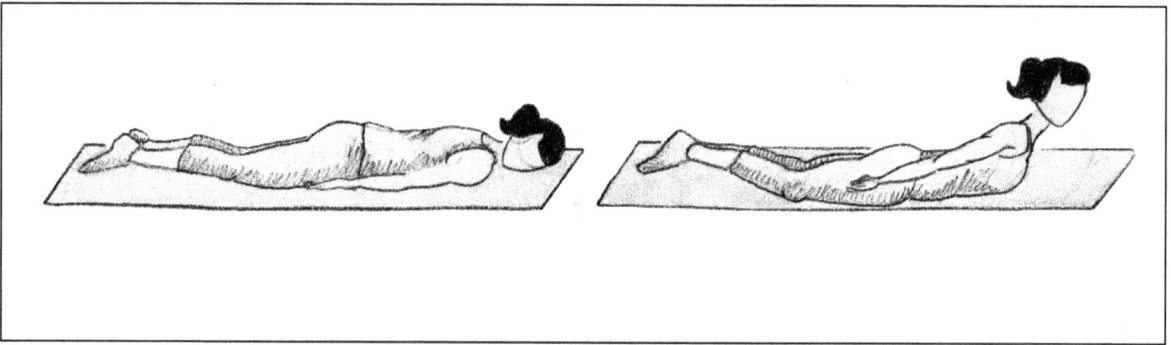

1) Lie on your stomach with your arms at your sides and palms facing up.

2) Slowly raise your front shoulders up off the ground by contracting your lower back.

3) Simultaneously, raise your toes off the ground.

4) Do three sets of 20 repetitions. Don't hyperextend your back.

Some additional tips for preventing and getting rid of Muffin Tops:

> Have patience. I always say fat around the waistline is like a bad in-law, it's the first to arrive and the last to leave. Your body is going to start taking fat away from other areas first, but know that once it's done that it targets the fat around the waistline. So keep your motivation and dedication going.

> Think about the magic number 3,500. One pound of weight loss equals 3,500 calories. So a pound per week equals 500 calories per day. Start looking at how you can shave off 500 calories per day, either by exercising longer to expend 500 calories, or by eating better to intake 500 calories less, or a combination of 250 calories each, which is a great choice.

Staying Motivated and Engaged

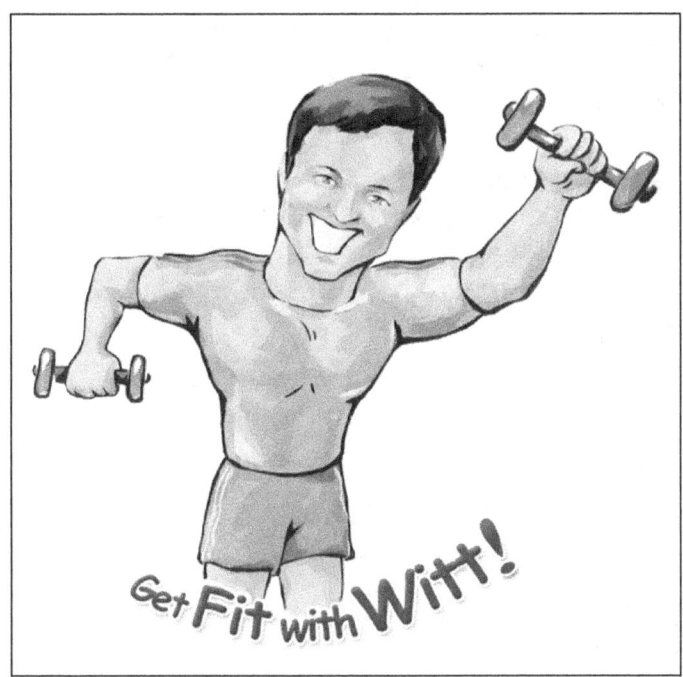

There are going to be a lot of distractions, obstacles, and barriers to your success along the way when getting rid of Cankles, Bat Wings, Thunder Thighs, and Muffin Tops, and more. So when you "fall off the wagon," here's how to pick yourself back up and resume your forward momentum, taking charge of your health and wellness.

Forget Perfection

First of all, always remember that you are not perfect, and that even fitness professionals like me have bad days where we slip on our diet or our exercise. The most important thing to do is simply "take two." Remember how I talked about this being the movie of your life, starring YOU and also directed by YOU? So if you slip up and overeat or skip a workout session, just remember your movie has a big budget and you can re-shoot the scene the next day for a second take. Don't beat yourself up, just take "action" and get back in the scene and give an award winning performance the next day.

Look Beyond the Cosmetic Effects

Second, go beyond the cosmetic benefits of exercising and eating right. About two weeks into your program, start to write down and record other benefits such as, "feel more flexible," or, "more energy and endurance at work," or even, "sleeping better now." After adopting a healthier lifestyle, the benefits to you will be numerous, each one building on a previous benefit until pretty soon it's a snowball effect of good things.

Here are just some of the things I've heard over the years from my clients after they've taken charge of their health and wellness:

- "Less stiffness and pain in joints"
- "Better mental focus and clarity"
- "Able to manage stressors better"
- "Stronger and more flexible"
- "I'm simply happier"
- "Improvement in biomarkers"
- "Better range of motion"
- "Less headaches"
- "Better eyesight"
- "More self confidence"
- "Improved bone density"
- "Easier pregnancy and birth"
- "Reduction in T-cell count"
- "Weight loss"
- "Body fat loss"
- "Improved performance for sports"
- "Cure diabetes"
- "Better balance "
- "Less heartburn and acid reflux"
- "Feel the need to drink less alcohol"
- "Less sickness with flu and colds "
- "Breathe easier"
- "More sociable"
- "Quality time with kids"
- "Able to volunteer more"
- "More spiritual"
- "Stronger faith"
- "Urge to pursue my dreams"

And the list goes on and on and on and on and on and on! Kind of seems too good to be true, doesn't it? Well, it isn't. I've seen and witnessed all this for the past 10 years through my business, GetFitwithWitt.com!

Some other benefits are: the longer you remain consistent with maintaining an exercise program and good eating habits, the more efficient your body will become at burning off its fat stores for an energy source during exercise. Your body relies on stored carbohydrates (glycogen stored in the body) for energy, too, especially for more intense, shorter-duration exercises. Lower intensity, longer-duration exercises tend to utilize more of your fat stores for energy, so here you can see how jogging, hiking, or biking can be a great way to start to train your body to use fat for fuel. Once that starts happening, when you do more intense shorter-duration workouts such as resistance training, your body becomes better at switching over to fat for fuel.

Also, as we age our muscle mass starts to decrease, which makes our metabolism slow down (metabolism is our body's ability to convert food and other substances into energy, essentially its calorie burning ability). In particular, this becomes a real issue for people over the age of 50. Strength and resistance type of exercises help to retain as much of your muscle mass as possible, therefore keeping your metabolism elevated. Always remember a pound of fat on your body only burns about 2 to 3 calories per day, whereas a pound of lean skeletal muscle burns roughly 50 calories per day. Can you see the difference it can make as you replace your body fat with lean skeletal muscle tissue? Your body becomes a lean, mean calorie burning machine, even while you are watching TV and sleeping!

Putting It All Together

So there you have it, folks, a way to take charge of your health and well being while also getting rid of those pesky problem areas on your body, to look and feel your best every single day. I implore you to, "Stop Making Excuses, Focus, and Do Something About It." SMEFADSAI, SMEFADSAI, SMEFADSAI!!

What are you going to do tomorrow to strengthen your emotional intelligence? Create a network of support and friends? How about your faith in fitness? And what about your ability to just immerse yourself into this and get a little bit crazy?

Stay focused on all of these by keeping a journal highlighting each day's SMEDFADSAI and the benefits you are starting to realize from your exercise and diet program. Perhaps a blog would be ideal for you, or a daily status update on Facebook, or even a Pinterest pin. Organize your life from here on out, to keep you focused, informed, and motivated to becoming the real YOU.

The fitness road ahead isn't going to be easy, there are going to be barriers and obstacles that you will need to overcome and get past. One of biggest challenges I hear from people these days is that they think they don't have TIME. The bottom line on this one, you absolutely have to make and carve out the time somehow. This is your life, your health, your wellness, and your happiness. You have to be able to find at least 30 minutes a day for moderate to strenuous physical activity. Get up earlier, do two 15-minute exercise sessions throughout the day, cut down on TV and computer time in order to fit in an exercise session, etc. The TIME thing can't be an excuse; it's just not acceptable.

Another big obstacle I see clients struggle with is food management. Again, this is in my opinion 70% of becoming healthy and in shape. Don't let it discourage you if you fall off track one day and overeat. Just resume again on your path to health and wellness and try to counter the bad day by eating extra good foods the next day. It's a constant balancing act with food, nobody eats perfectly, but as long as you counter any bad behaviors with a resulting extremely good behavior, you should be fine. It's when you stay off course and revert back to a "give up" attitude that you fail to open the door for the real YOU to blossom.

Healthy, Fun and Easy Recipes

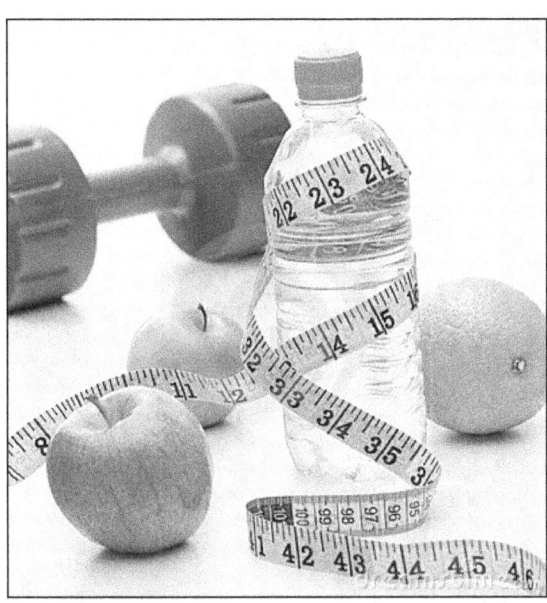

Mojgan's Heirloom Tomato Truffle Salad

Chunks of 2 color tomatoes, chunks of watermelons/any melon (steak thickness cut). Drizzle with nice vinaigrette and truffle oil.

Susan's Hummus Egg Cups

Take a boiled egg, cut in half and ditch the yoke, fill the egg white cups with hummus - a high protein pick me up with very low calories.

Susan's Greek Yogurt/Salsa Dip

Mix one individual size non-fat green yogurt cup with hot/spicy prepared salsa, to taste.

Pair dip with: carrots, sliced Persian cucumbers, or red pepper slices.

You'll get your protein, veggies and spices (good for inflammation).

Anna's Cucumber Soup

(Serves 4)

Ingredients:

1 lb long cucumbers, peeled and coarsely grated
1 garlic clove, crushed
1 tsp ground cumin
2 cups unsweetened natural yogurt
1/2 cup vegetable stock + extra in reserve
Salt
3 tbsp chopped pistachios, for serving
3 tbsp dill sprigs, for serving

Instructions:

Blend cucumber, garlic, cumin and yogurt in a food processor until smooth.

Transfer to a mixing bowl and stir in stock, adding more if soup is too thick. Season to taste.

Cover soup and refrigerate for at least 30 minutes to chill. Serve soup topped with pistachios and dill.

The Get Fit with Witt ! Mid-afternoon Power Punchin' Pick-me-Upper

In a large bowl place:

1 sliced medium banana
1 cup of plain Nonfat Greek Yogurt
2 tablespoons of All-Natural Unsalted Smooth Peanut Butter
1 tablespoon of Raw-Wild Natural Honey

Sprinkle on top (sparingly) some Grape Nuts cereal to give it a crunch.

Annie's Favorite Greek Yogurt Snack

1 carton (6oz) Fahe Greek nonfat yogurt
1 tbspn low calorie fruit jam (25-35 calories)
Handful of raisins, blueberries or diced fresh fruit

1 tbspn chopped or sliced almonds, peanuts, walnuts or pecans

1 tbspn granola

Cinnamon and nutmeg to taste.

First blend yogurt and jam, then add remaining ingredients, and sprinkle the spices on last.

Lifestyle Insights Reports

"It's an Owner's Manual for your Body & Mind"

One of my staple products throughout the years to help people take charge of their health and wellness is my "Lifestyle Insights Report," an owner's manual for your body and mind that you can refer back to for the rest of your life, because it's created for YOU by YOU!

Here's how it works: You'll take a quick 10-minute assessment online, which will generate a customized 18-page report that will pave the way toward your self-discovery. Lifestyle Insights will help you stop stressors before they happen, break bad habits, tap into your personal energy, and get truly motivated to make positive changes in your life. You'll get to know yourself better, understand how your body's inter-related systems affect you, and gain valuable insight into your own unique behavior style. The Lifestyle Insights system will then help you create a 30-day action plan, based on your personal self-discovery process.

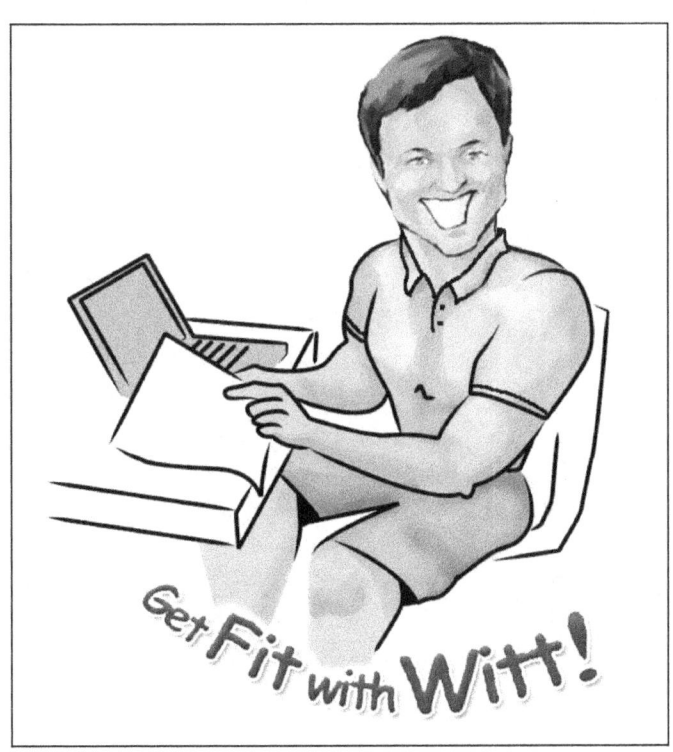

It's important to understand that if your natural and adapted styles don't match, you are probably under too much stress and pressure, by putting your "mask" on every day. With *Lifestyle Insights Reports* you will gain an understanding of your individual style, including insight into your strengths and weaknesses, so that you can reach your full potential.

Order your Lifestyle Insights Report today for only $99 - which includes your Lifestyle Insights Report, Self Guided Workbook, along with additional online tools. As a Professional Certified Behavioral Analyst, I'm personally available to guide you through a 60-minute intensive telephone debriefing session for an additional $59.

You can view a sample report and purchase your *Lifestyle Insights Report* on my website at GetFitwithWitt.com or email me directly at Jack@GetFitwithWitt.com.

Special Thanks and Dedication

Kaitlin Howell - for the fun and retro looking illustrations to go along with these books.

Leslie Le Mon - for her coaching and feedback along every step of the way of the journey of writing and publishing my first book(s). Email her at les.lemon.author@gmail.com as she is always happy to consult with writers, first-time or otherwise.

Cherie Higgins - for proofing the book(s).

All my personal fitness training clients throughout the years who would come up to me from time to time and ask me how to get rid of these certain fatty, flabby and out of shape areas on our bodies, and called them by the funny names referenced in the book title. You guys absolutely set the wheels in motion for these books! *Stefanie, Lisa, Ilene & Jim & Sylvia, Alda, Kara & both Davids, Eric, Cookie, Erwin, Mark, Youchanan, Jim, Betsy, Anna, Tanya, Paulina, Selenne, Sonia, Annie!, Kirk, Aliki, Leanne, Jeanne, Jane & Keith, Tony & Lana, Sheila, Gloria, Elizabeth, Lisa, Ellen* and *Elaine, Lisa* and *Nancy* and *Jessica, Jane & Dorain, Susan, Emily, Thang & Nancy, Paul, Lou, David, Sean, Kimberly, Annie, Kevin, Scott, Stacy* and *Matt, Phil, Elaine (Ink), Stephanie, King, Donna, Michael, Jaime* and *Jackie, Chris, CherylAnn, Stuart &Robin, Jane & Dorain, MaryLu, Karen & Karen & Andreas, Roz, Ricky, Beneranda, Mayra, Breanna, Sylvia, Mojgan, Patricia, Gina & Dezi & Anna, Bill, Marlene & Chris, Roni* and *Tess, Stuart & Robyn, Zaven, Justin, Kristie, LuLu, Trudy,* and *Howard.*

Greg Highley - for my personal photographs.

Rony Armas & Agnes Avagyan - for the cartoon Jacks.

Adisorn "Tan" Toonsap - for photo editing.

Carrie Spencer - for Webmastering.

The personal fitness training gyms that I've worked with over the years, including *BodyImage, AtOneFitness, BodyUSA, ShapeIt,* and *Knuckles.*

Some of the other super great fitness trainers I've had the opportunity to work on community and charity projects with over the years – *Nancy Sexton, Steven Greene, Lisa Smith* and *Wendie Wilson.*

NohoArtsDistrict.com - for allowing me the forum to blog and write about fitness and health, and in which I first introduced explanations and exercises for many of these funny named problem body areas.

The *California Jaycees* and the *UCNH Chamber of Commerce* - for invaluable experience helping to build my leadership and business skills, as well as my network of community contacts; many of whom still train with me to this day. And the other community groups I've had the pleasure to build healthy community with, such as *The North Hollywood Rotary, North Hollywood/Studio City Kiwanis, Encino Chamber, North Hollywood High School Key Club* and *NoHo Communications Group*.

One of my very first clients, *Stefanie Ibanez* - for coming up with my business tag line/name: *"Get Fit with Witt!"* Shout it out, people!!

SADA Systems - for developing and managing my website and hosting.

The late *Deby Harper* - for introducing me to *Lifestyle Insights* and helping me personally discover more about myself.

This book is dedicated to one of the most beloved baseball and football little league coaches out of Northeast Ohio; my Dad, *Jack Howard Witt*. He taught us kids to play fair, not to underestimate ourselves or what we could achieve as a team, and to be proud of who we are. RIP, Coach!

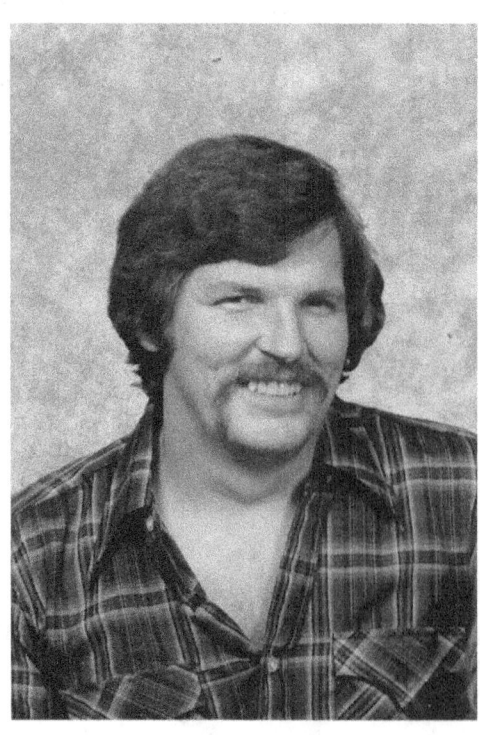

About the Author

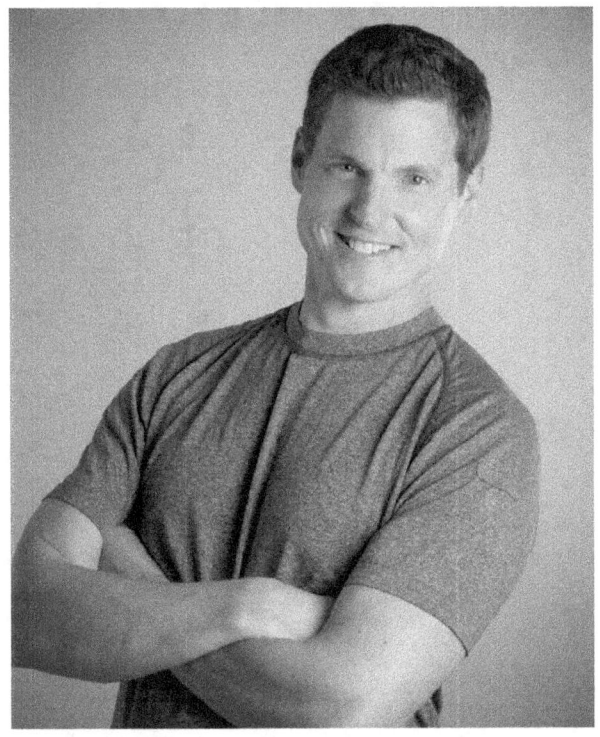

Jack Witt is a health and fitness coach, based out of Los Angeles since 2003. He holds a Master's Degree in Exercise Science, and is a healthy community organizer, serving as past President of the Universal City North Hollywood Jaycees (Junior Chamber) and Chamber of Commerce. His awards include "Outstanding Young Californian", "Angel" and "Small Business of the Year."

He is an NASM Certified Personal Fitness Trainer and TTI Certified Behavioral Analyst. His public speaking and workshop engagements include Los Angeles Unified School District, Social Security Administration, Volunteer League of the San Fernando Valley, and Los Angeles Valley College. Jack has worked with kids, adults and seniors, helping all of them take charge of their health and wellness.

Visit Jack's website at: www.GetfitwithWitt.com

Follow Jack on Twitter @GetfitwithWitt

Subscribe to Jack's YouTube Channel at:
http://www.youtube.com/user/getfitwithWitt

Copyrights

All content, illustrations, and photos in *Tight, Tone and Trim: How to get rid of Cankles, Bat Wings, Thunder Thighs, and Muffin Tops. And much, much more!,* including the cover design; are created by, property of, and copyrighted by Jack Witt © 2013. Healthy Recipe Photo Source: Google Images. Exercise instructions inspired by FitnessGenerator.com.